The Handbook of Intermittent Fasting

Effective Solutions for Muscle Definition & Weight Loss

By Idai Makaya

ISBN 978-1-4452-0454-3   *Copyright © Idai Makaya 2009*

Contents

Caution: *Intermittent Fasting is not to be used during pregnancy and cannot be used by persons under 18 years old - although it can be used post-pregnancy (after clearance by a qualified healthcare professional). Please consult your family doctor before commencing **any** exercise or eating program and if you suffer from a chronic or temporary health condition it is essential that you first have a medical check-up and get clearance to proceed. The advice given here must be evaluated by the reader and should not substitute medical advice from your doctor.*

Please Note:

I recommend that anyone who decides to take up any new eating or exercise practice (certainly if it is based around fasting) does so under experienced supervision. Although the eating protocols to be outlined here will suit the overwhelming majority of people it is important to be aware of the fact that the initial transition to a fasting protocol is likely to differ between individuals and some individuals will not be able to recognise – or distinguish between – some of the expected changes and other (unexpected) events which may occur during this time.

In addition, eating-disorders must be legislated for whenever engaging in activities related to weight-loss and it makes sense to be medically cleared for one's own safety and protection.

All the issues alluded to above will be addressed in this book.

Introduction

Intermittent Fasting (IF) is the process of using **scheduled** and **controlled** sessions/periods of food **restriction** to effect fat loss and improved health. The term has not been strictly defined but for purposes of the protocols to be outlined here these **fasting sessions need never exceed 24 hours in duration** (typically, they range in length from 16 to 24 hours). This handbook aims to inform readers of the benefits and advantages of intermittent fasting and to share my own experiences of using different techniques to attain a leaner, more defined physique - or to lose weight.

Please make due consideration for your own fitness and health status when contemplating the use of a new dietary plan, such as IF - and if you have any underlying health-related conditions (whether **mental or physical**), you must consult with your healthcare specialist before and during your commencement phase.

Over recent years I have increasingly relied on the technique of IF to strip body fat and to lose weight - and in the latter half of 2008 I decided **I had gathered and found enough evidence to justify following IF protocols indefinitely (should the user so choose)**. Prior to 2008 I'd felt that I needed to see and examine more data about the long term **safety** prospects of IF (**efficacy** usually becomes obvious within just a few weeks). Also, I still needed to document my own personal experiences over a long enough period of time spent using different IF protocols and to have regular long term health checks to monitor and confirm my progress.

Having looked into these aspects of my own personal journey over a reasonable period of time I now feel I have been able to make an informed and scientific evaluation of mine and other people's IF experiences. **I am now fully convinced of the safety and efficacy of the practice**. For this reason I feel it is prudent that I put together this guide to IF protocols, which will help me share my learnings and also help others to discover IF best practices - without having to re-invent the wheel or follow a single, dogmatic approach.

I am certain now that the multiple-fixed-meal eating plan is a result of cultural (rather than biological) needs/preferences and that the multiple, frequent meal system has actually propagated the obesity crises commonplace in all developed countries and societies where there is predictable, accessible food supply for most of the population. Human bodies are designed for a life of unpredictable food supply and are thus designed to work best under frugal, intermittent/fluctuating food-supply conditions. There is little disagreement about this fact among all credible researchers and authorities (hence the repeated and unified calls to stem the Western obesity crisis).

When certain nutrients (which were normally rare in nature a few thousand years ago) become easily accessible - in unlimited quantities - the majority of people will (statistically) fail to maintain a stable weight, because we are designed to crave such nutrients in an unlimited fashion

and generally lack the mechanisms to deal with oversupply. In nature there is no risk of animals 'overdosing' on scarce minerals/nutrients, so animals are designed to crave these nutrients – without any limiting mechanisms to stop them from "over consuming" such foods (as the need to develop such mechanisms has never arisen – until now).

IF is a solution for dealing with the challenge of regulating our eating (and minimising our body fat). Later I will explain why the elimination of body fat is **not just a cosmetic undertaking**, but is crucial for allowing us to attain our full natural lifespan; without being hindered in that endeavour by cancer and other genetic, lifestyle-dependent diseases.

In conditions of unpredictable food supply, which most authorities agree the human body is developed for, one **cannot** guarantee numerous, predicted mealtimes. However, in society now we often see guaranteed oversupply and exposure to convenient, easily accessible on-demand food consumption.

There still needs to be a minimum frequency of food consumption required to maintain good health – eating is an unavoidable and necessary part of life and cannot be neglected! But this minimum necessary feeding frequency is much lower than the averages now common in prosperous modern societies. This is observed in all societies now with the same pathological outcomes. Even in the poorest countries in the world there are still "pockets" of prosperity, wealthy individuals who are able to access whatever they want. In those "pockets" the same pathologies observed in Western countries present in much the same way to threaten life expectancy via diseases and conditions such as the "metabolic syndrome" and cancer, etc.

Purposeful studies have shown this minimum meal frequency to be much lower than is commonly perceived. However, one need not aim for the minimum possible meal frequency - if comfort and enjoyment are still to be a part of everyday life. But we should still aim to manipulate this biological concept of meal frequency to our advantage - and that should be the aim of IF protocols.

IF is designed to allow for flexible eating patterns, which will suit both our weight control goals and our day to day lives. The only real reason why any genuine weight control eating method ever fails its users is **because it does not suit their lifestyles in a way that they can maintain long term. This handbook is designed to offer enough alternatives to allow the flexible use of IF over an indefinite period - so that inconvenience and lack of willpower do not intervene to impede progress with your weight maintenance goals.** If you can do this successfully over the long-term you will never have problems with unwanted body fat or weight control, ever again.

Like most physical culturalists – and even most of the general public – in the past I have found it difficult to reconcile the concept of fasting with good healthy eating practice - or athletic goals - and the transition towards a total reliance on IF has taken me quite a few years, mainly for this reason alone. **It** is my hope that this analysis of IF protocols will help others avoid the long journey I have been on and will put all the information they need to take up this highly beneficial practice into one place for easy access and reference.

Don't get me wrong - although I have personally never followed any kind of multiple-meal-weight-loss-diet (such as the 5 or 6 meals a day promoted by fitness magazines) for weight loss, I have no doubt that the system works. And the system works for the same reasons that IF works – calorie restriction. However, by nature, only a small minority of us will maintain a stable, ideal body weight using this practice. I still know of nobody who properly follows IF over a long period and is not very lean. However, only a few people in modern society are not 'soft bodied' following the traditional multiple meal strategy over the long term – especially in adult life. Accessibility of food has recently become so high in modern societies that the majority of citizens have lost the ability to control their bodyweight while following the traditional eating patterns prevalent in society. This has become a problem of epidemic proportions.

Multiple small meals are a strategy to restrict calories, while doing a small amount of feeding every time hunger beckons. It works, but it requires enormous discipline to fight the hunger promoted by following the method because **satiety is not really permitted under this system**. This is why so few people succeed in maintaining a lean bodyweight using the method. Those who do succeed do so though good discipline, but statistics show that the vast majority who try to achieve this will eventually fail (hence the obesity crisis we now face). The reason why most people fail on the traditional accepted eating plan is that it is actually unnatural (as already explained).

Before using IF my main strategy for weight loss was to create calorie deficits purely through a high volume of cardiovascular exercise. The method is valid and it works just as well as IF for fat burning purposes (in my personal experience and according to the science as well). However, it is not practical for everyone, all the time - and the birth of my first child in 2005 put this plainly into perspective for me.

I needed to create as much family time as I could in the time leading up to and just after the birth of my first child so I decided to switch from using a gym to using mainly home-based fitness training methods - something I have been very successful with developing. I also started looking at alternative ways of losing weight which would not require regular long hours of cardiovascular training on most days of the week. I now exercise 2 or 3 times a week, for about half an hour each session and I use IF to burn fat - instead of additional cardio sessions just for weight loss. The only cardio I do now is directly related to fitness and sports training and is not intended purely to induce weight loss. I believe exercise is good for conditioning and fitness and diet is **more practical** for controlling weight than high exercise volumes.

I am confident that full health and fitness can be maintained on just one weekly exercise session (if it is correctly structured to meet all fitness needs and if the exercises are sequenced in the appropriate order) **and just one meal a day** (if it is structured correctly to meet nutritional demands and contains sufficient calories to sustain energy demands for the individual concerned). This is a practice I have followed myself on numerous occasions and for lengthy periods (when it has suited my prevailing situation) and it is actually relatively easily sustainable. However, it best suits people with enormous time constraints and various work or family demands and is probably less enjoyable for most people than other IF protocols (which are possibly almost equally effective).

IF is actually quite natural, as explained earlier – and I will add more detail to this concept in later chapters. There are currently a number of IF protocols being used around the world and a number of reliable authorities on the topic who promote the various versions of the practice. However, many of the authorities on IF, to whom I refer above, have become very dogmatic about **which** particular approaches should be used – usually to the total exclusion of practices not promoted by themselves (something common in many fields of human endeavour and understandable for those and for financial reasons).

However, like most forms of human endeavour, there are many genuine routes to success and most people can find a variation - or hybridisation - of IF options which will suit their individual circumstances perfectly. Likewise, the more effective one's methodology becomes, the fewer the options available for excellence. For this reason, you will find that **there are really 3 or 4 major variants of IF - and all the other options are merely hybrids of these variants.**

This book aims to outline those basic pillars of IF philosophy and to then offer a methodology for finding an exact hybrid to suit your own personal circumstances (users of IF must realise that it is important to stick to your methodology for about 6 months before considering alterations - although it is good practice to make regular progress checks and to make a mini-evaluation of efficacy after about 3 months on a protocol). Monitoring of weight and body measurements is a good way of doing this. I will explain how best to do this later in this book.

Weight loss can be achieved through many means, but there are some common rules to all methods. Two of the foundation rules of weight loss **(by any method)** are as follows:

1. **You cannot expect to lose more than 1 kilo - or about 2 pounds - of fat in a single week (on average).** If you lose weight faster than this, the weight loss will also include muscle or water loss. This template should be used to set **all weight loss targets/goals** and will allow you to determine how long it will take you to reach your **ideal bodyweight** (ideal bodyweight will be defined later in this book).
2. **To lose weight you must consume fewer calories (or burn more calories) than you currently do.** You cannot lose weight **without creating a deficit in calories.** A deficit in calories refers to your body burning more energy than it is taking in, over a period of time. **This**

also implies, logically, that you cannot lose weight indefinitely - or you'll die of starvation. This concept also logically dictates that **eventually all weight loss must stop** and a **weight-loss program must eventually be abandoned**.

The abandonment of a weight loss program need not mean reverting to uncontrolled weight gain. One must endeavour to keep body fat low at all times, but it is important to realise that a **weight maintenance plan** must be commenced once all excess weight is lost. **IF can serve in both capacities – weight loss and weight maintenance**. In the past I have used IF mainly for weight loss and then stopped the practice until a predetermined weight gain limit was reached once more. This, I believe, was as a result of the last vestiges of the common diet concept prevalent in physical culture, sports and fitness - whereby individuals reach a body fat goal and then back off for a while, until they have regained weight.

I think **the practice is reasonable - as long as one doesn't allow too much weight regain**. However, for purposes of the wider population demographic and general community health, I have reached the conclusion that it's best to focus on permanent programs for weight loss and then maintenance - and I will be focusing my efforts mostly on lifestyle modifications (rather than short term, intense programs) in this book. That way, my recommendations will be more suitable for the majority of people.

I believe it is a good idea to annually strip off all the excess body fat you've gained over the prior year(s) for health and detoxification reasons - and this is something I have done every year for much of my adult life, through various means. So even if you do not choose to use IF permanently, do keep focus on stripping off all excess fat every year for the rest of your life, even if you allow some weight gain to then recur. The reasons why fat stripping works for detoxification are explained a little later in this document, but the main focus of this book will be the achievement of one's ideal bodyweight - with good muscle definition - attained through the use of an intermittent fasting protocol.

Intermittent Fasting Defined

*Intermittent Fasting (IF for short) is a means of controlled abstention from eating for **predetermined**, **scheduled** periods.* Note the emphasis on "predetermined" and "scheduled." The scheduling of this "fasting" must be adhered to over lengthy periods of time and it must fit specific criteria to be defined as "healthy."

For clarity I will outline the criteria for "healthy" fasting below:

1. Healthy fasting **follows a predetermined plan**. **Planning** is an essential feature of healthy fasting.
2. Healthy fasting is **used to attain a predetermined ideal bodyweight** (I will explain how this determination can be made). If you fast to the extent that you drop under the "ideal" bodyweight for your height and build you have an eating disorder. If you fast with no idea of when minimum weight has been reached I think it indicates a problem as well. Healthy fasting must enforce calorie restriction/control while still paying full attention to **nutritional balance – you must follow an ideally balanced diet.** This is even more important in a diet with restricted calories than it is for someone who overeats (because you get a smaller window of opportunity to get your nutrient balance right when you consume fewer calories). If you knowingly become malnourished you probably have an eating disorder – regardless of how much you actually eat.

If you decide to fast healthily you must stick to these criteria - or else what you are actually doing is developing an eating disorder. I know there is a fine line between eating disorders and "diets" but I do not think IF is any riskier than any other means of eating/dieting to lose weight - in relation to developing eating disorders. What is really important in the avoidance of such eating disorders is good mental health and a full understanding of what you are trying to achieve - and how it can be achieved.

Ignorance, mental stress (or mental instability) and a lack of defined weight loss goals are the main risk factors for developing eating disorders. This is a subject everyone who tries to manipulate his/her weight needs to be aware of.

IF is classified as a **Calorie Restriction (CR for short)** weight loss diet or lifestyle. The implication is that the benefits of intermittent fasting for weight loss are derived from the control of calories taken in over a period of time. This is generally true, although IF seems to have additional benefits beyond those associated with weight loss – even in the absence of calorie restriction.

This book will outline the various benefits associated with the practice of intermittent fasting and will also offer different protocols for performing intermittent fasting. Like most healthy practices, intermittent fasting is best used as part of a positive lifestyle alteration - and not merely for short spells of time. In order to do this, it is necessary to have a wide variety of flexible options to choose from and to create potential variety in the routine.

The main reason for this variety is that the mind (and sometimes the body) often requires regular breaks from routine in order to maintain good responses to progressive stimuli. You don't want to become mentally stale and variety in routine can often help avoid this. With intermittent fasting, changes in routine are not absolutely necessary – and even for those who like variety in routine (such as myself), such changes need not be implemented more regularly than every few months.

The advantage of having a number of protocols to use is that you can try out the different routines over a period of time to find which ones work best for your particular body - and it also offers flexibility so that you can maintain your routine despite any changes in regular day to day activities or circumstances.

The Link between Your Weight and Muscle Definition

It is important at this stage to define (pardon the pun) the concept of muscle definition. Muscle definition is purely a visual effect, whereby the muscles of the physique are easily discernible in both shape and individuality – basically a lean appearance.

There are two main contributing factors to achieving this appearance and it is important to be aware of these. **One factor is the amount of fat under the skin. The other is the size and development of the muscles themselves.**

Without the manipulation of both these factors, simultaneously, a defined appearance is impossible. Fat must be minimal and muscles should be reasonably developed to result in the appearance of a lean, defined physique.

Other additional factors influencing muscle definition are water content under the skin and the complexion of the skin – high water content under the skin will obscure the visibility of the underlying muscles and darker skin shows definition better due to contrast caused by the bulged muscle shapes.

This correctly implies that the only way to attain a defined appearance is to develop the muscles and minimise the amount of fat on your body. This is the basis of using intermittent fasting to improve muscle definition and (correctly) implies that intermittent fasting should really be used alongside a strength training program to develop the muscles.

Defined muscles need **not** be very large. However, they must be developed to an extent that they have a discernible shape. Conversely, it is impossible to define your body without minimising your body fat – regardless of muscular size and definition.

Most people have bodies which can be easily sculpted **for aesthetic purposes** - but the more fat one carries under the skin, the larger the muscles have to become in order to still be noticed through the fat. Be aware also of the fact that regardless of how little fat you have on your body, without some moderate muscular development you will still not appear to be defined or sculpted. Good examples of the latter concept are elite marathon runners who have virtually no body fat but still do not appear defined on the upper body, because they do not do any strength training and have minimal muscular development of the upper body. Good examples of the former concept are heavyweight power lifters who appear to be fat, despite obviously well developed muscles (hidden deep beneath the fat).

I hope these analogies and explanations have convinced readers of the concepts integral to obtaining muscle definition. I think this distinction is important to make because the majority of people I come across who want to improve their muscle definition seem to think they can do so by simply toiling away at certain exercises, relentlessly, in the hope that one day their muscle definition will improve through muscular development alone. However, that strategy only works for people whose body fat is already extremely low.

Having said this, a good general exercise program, focused on strength training and cardiovascular/aerobic exercise will yield a healthier body, which is better able to metabolise fat (and, thus, become even leaner). It is also worth noting that weight loss through calorie restriction (**of any kind**) can cause muscles to be broken down for energy purposes, if "protein sparing" mechanisms are not stimulated.

"Protein sparing" refers to the body selectively metabolising fat for energy and avoiding breakdown of the proteins in the muscles. The best ways to stimulate this effect (according to scientific studies) are to train the muscles to become stronger and fitter - and to intermittently fast. However, at extremes of calorie restriction, muscles may still be broken down, especially in the absence of the exercise stimulus. So **exercise is a crucial part of weight loss because it ensures fat is broken down - and not the muscles, instead**.

The next chapter will look at the concept of calorie restriction (CR) and will explain the benefits of this practice – linking those to the benefits of intermittent fasting in general.

The Benefits of Intermittent Fasting

The most obvious benefit of IF, when used correctly, is weight loss. You are more likely to lose weight (and maintain your ideal weight) using intermittent fasting than by other means of regulating your food intake, because the defined boundaries set for eating (and not eating) are more clearly drawn out in IF. The key advantage of IF is it's suitability as an easier (hence, long term) weight control solution.

At this point you will probably be asking how I can justify such a statement and I will do so now. IF sets clear boundaries for calorie restriction - you either eat, or you abstain - based on the dictates of your IF program. If, for instance, you were to follow a daily fasting program, eating within a 4 hour window period every day, you would know that you cannot take in calories outside the eating window period, so you would not need to deliberate/debate about whether you should – or shouldn't - be tempted by the chocolate bar you see at a shop till; or by the biscuits brought in for tea during your business meeting, etc.

The rules are clear and that takes away the conflict. Also, IF doesn't place mandatory restrictions on **what** you are allowed to eat - within reason (this allows you to curb cravings because **no food is permanently off bounds**, although certain less-healthy foods should be minimised, according to the dictates of good nutrition). On the other hand, if you are on a diet which instructs you to limit what you eat by eating less of everything - **across the entire day** - or hardly ever eating certain other things - the debate is blown out of proportion whenever you have to categorise any specific temptation that may arise. The reality of this concept is much more profound than it would sound to the uninitiated and it is a powerful concept in practice.

The margin for error is constrained during IF because you only need to be on the alert (and making these decisions) for a very short period of time each day. **The rest of the time, there is no debate about eating - the rules are clearer. It is a purely statistical thing** - if you only need to be diligent for 4 hours out of every 24 hours, then **you are 6 times more likely to succeed** in your diet than someone who needs to be vigilant for all 24 hours. When using IF you still need to follow a 'diet' of sorts, during the eating periods - but the controlled length of these periods restricts any potential 'damage' bad choices may potentially inflict.

All good lifestyle changes should appeal to "the child within us." This refers to our subconscious minds. When a child knows certain things are totally off bounds, you will notice that the child will not try to bargain with his/her parents for those things. But if those 'things' are sometimes allowed, and sometimes not, it becomes more difficult to control a child who doesn't understand **why** those permissions apply. This is very much how the subconscious mind works. **Work with your subconscious mind rather than**

against it because you will eventually fail if you try to ignore the pull of the subconscious.

This is because you'll fail to address those subconscious food choice debates whenever they arise, which will intensify their significance in the subconscious perspective. However, by addressing them in a way that fits in with the way the subconscious mind works, **you can keep the subconscious mind permanently at bay**. But the rules **must** be observed – **appeal to the 'inner child.'**

You don't need to test your willpower by trying to limit and regulate your eating through sheer willpower alone when using IF, because manageable periods of discipline are balanced with periods of reasonable laxity. The balancing of disciplined periods with periods of laxity gives a regular sense of achievement and control - which gives sense of motivation as well.

I strongly believe that dietary programs focussed around constant discipline - with very little scheduled laxity - are too rigid to serve as lifestyle changes for 70% of the population. 30% can do it, but most cannot. This is my justification for the effectiveness of IF in the long term. Of course, this implies implementing IF correctly, if you do not follow the rules to be outlined in this manual you may find some forms of IF difficult to do. Please adhere to the rules and logic so that the various programs can actually work for you.

There are other less-obvious potential benefits to be derived as well. These have been seen in various human and animal studies and will be discussed below:

- **Extended life spans** are the most obvious benefit of CR and IF regimes. Research on animals (with life spans short enough to be observed repeatedly across many generations in scientific laboratories) shows that application of intermittent fasting protocols to animals' lives results in great extensions of their life spans (upwards of 30%). This is regarded as a common effect of **calorie restriction**. However, it has been shown that these benefits can still be derived from IF **even when calories are not actually restricted and weight is not lost. This suggests that IF has advantages beyond just those of calorie restriction.** More work needs to be done to fully explain this phenomenon, but the hypothesis which most likely accounts for the effect is that **fasting periods activate certain genes**, which cause the animals' cells to proliferate and replace themselves more slowly and, hence, to maintain themselves longer. **Ageing is, thus, slowed by fasting – even without any weight loss or calorie restriction**. As I mentioned previously, this has so far been seen in animal studies and is not fully understood **(human lifespan studies take generations, so we will not know how well this effect of IF manifests in the human model – unless we take the voyage of discovery ourselves)**.
- The closest anecdotal examples of life-extension through fasting are seen in the **Eastern Yogis**, who are often recorded as being over 100 years old. Many of them claim to be well over 100 years old and are

still in good shape, but these claims often cannot be verified. My personal approach to lifespan is that we are not intended to live forever - but **quality of life is important**. If we do things that will extend our lifespan, then we are giving ourselves the best chances of having a high **quality** of life, relatively free from disease and infirmity. **Because life is often about cause and effect** - it is erroneous to believe that everything happens purely by luck. **IF is a means of taking more control over your life, its potential length and its potential quality.** We have choices available in our lives (no matter how small these choices may or may not be) which will enable us to influence the eventual courses and outcomes of our lives. IF is one such choice.

- There are also many **short term benefits of IF** which have been studied thoroughly - such as its massive **impact on cholesterol and lipid profiles** and the improvement of the symptoms of type 2 diabetes (as a result of the increased insulin sensitivity brought about by fasting). Fasting appears to have similar effects on **increasing insulin sensitivity** as increased exercise does - in sedentary people. The message here is to exercise and fast more often for better health and in order to avoid obesity-related type 2 diabetes.

- **Detoxification** refers to the fact that most toxins are stored in animals' body fat. This is why fatty meat should be avoided/moderated - and so should the visible fat on meat. The vast majority of toxins reside in the fat tissue and by breaking fat down free fatty acids are released into the bloodstream, to serve as an alternative fuel to glucose (sugar), for running the body. But alongside these fatty acids, all the stored toxins in the fat tissue are also released into the bloodstream and they then become available for excretion. **This process is at its height during a fast and this is the benefit of regular fasting - even for those who do not need to lose any weight. You can fast - and still avoid a calorie deficit - if you do not need to lose weight; but you'll still benefit from the fasting period.** This has been proved repeatedly in animal studies. Human life spans are too long to allow us to see the full effect this practice has on the human lifespan, but it is probably safe to assume it will be similar (as other short term benefits seen in animal studies seem to correlate with human studies). **It is primarily for this reason that most "Detox" programs have an element of fasting as their backbone.** The fasting common in Detox programs is intended to break down the fat tissues and the potions and soups, etc, consumed are intended to remove toxins from the bloodstream, when they are liberated.

- **Reduction in harmful enzymes** produced by fat (especially abdominal visceral fat). The more fat on the body, the higher the production of these enzymes (some of which have not yet been identified - or isolated - but are postulated to exist). Overproduction of these enzymes is responsible for what is now commonly termed the "metabolic syndrome," which includes the development of deadly health conditions such as diabetes, heart disease and cancer.

- **Activation of life-extending genes** seems to be another result of regular fasting periods and this is believed to be as a result of the fact that those genes have developed specifically to help animals survive well under conditions of unpredictable food supply. These are the **genes thought to influence susceptibility to cancer and metabolic diseases** and this effect also **ties in with the detoxification effect** of fasting – **toxins are often blamed for increased susceptibility to cancers and metabolic diseases**.

It appears these genes may also affect protein sparing mechanisms because most IF studies on animals (and people) suggest **a gain in lean muscle mass occurs in IF users, regardless of whether or not exercise protocols are simultaneously used**. The reason the genetic hypothesis would make sense in these cases of muscle gain is that starvation periods require enhanced "foraging," over extended ranges, for animals to find scarce food in a famine situation - so **it would make sense to preserve the machinery (muscles) needed to effect this**.

Further support of the genetic hypothesis is the fact that animals that die of starvation, although totally emaciated, often do not lose the ability to forage until just a few hours before the point of death. They are usually able to walk right up to within a few hours of when they eventually collapse and die. This suggests death under such circumstances is more a result of finally running out of the energy used to fuel the body and its vital functions (or death through malnutrition-induced disease). So it appears that death by starvation is not about total cannibalisation of muscle tissue and this extreme example serves to suggest a specific genetic design in animals has been developed to preserve muscle under times of food scarcity (or unpredictable supply).

The research also appears to suggest that regular periods of abstinence from food quickly alert the body to become more cautious about muscle breakdown due to uncertainty of food supply. Sticking to the same example, it appears these **"abstinences" from food should be of limited duration** because food restriction quickly leads to some muscle breakdown if it persists for too long. This is why the 24-32 hour maximum fasting time limit is imposed in most acceptable IF programs.

Some readers may ask what the **mechanism** of this enhanced gene expression is. At this point it is difficult to say exactly which factors play a role but one known factor is **the increased secretion of growth hormone under fasted conditions. Fasting increases growth hormone secretion** - in much the same way as exercise does - and this would account for the enhanced protein sparing observed in fasting (and even starving) organisms. Growth hormone secretions also explain the increased burning of fat as the preferred fuel source during fasting. Fat burning involves the release of the free fatty acids which make up fat cells and it liberates toxins to make them available for excretion (hence, the reduced risk for metabolic diseases and cancers). This response seems to be genetically mediated.

- **Regular resting of the digestive system** and cleansing of poor bacterial cultures from it is an obvious result of fasting. This is thought to be the reason why the first reaction of the body towards fighting serious illness and infections is to eliminate appetite. This frees energy to boost the immune system (as digestion is a very expensive process, energetically and biologically). Some health experts have developed disease-curing programs based solely on long fasts to improve immune system diseases. **The body is better able to repair and regulate itself under controlled fasted conditions.**

- **Energy levels** are actually boosted by fasting. Studies have now shown that people who panic and seem to feel awful when they go without food for a few hours are actually mainly suffering from psychological distress (and their blood sugar levels actually remain relatively stable). **Part of the adaptation to fasting is psychological.** This is not to say there isn't a physical adaptation involved (there certainly is - and it takes about a month). During the month of adjusting to fasting, some new users of the practice may feel uncomfortable and, often, very little weight is lost. But once the enzyme production processes have adapted the body becomes better at switching to running on fatty acids and secreting less insulin as a result. The sensitivity of cells to insulin also increases under those conditions, so that less insulin causes more glucose absorption than before the adaptation. This is a healthier metabolic state and helps to keep fat levels low (insulin increases weight gain so lower levels encourage fat burning and growth hormone secretion, which promotes protein sparing and muscle retention). **These effects are potentiated by the inclusion of regular exercise.** The outcome of regular fasting is greatly improved energy levels and lifted mood, especially during the actual fasting periods.

Again, the science behind improved energy levels and elevated mood during fasting probably links back to the genetic effects of fasting, mentioned earlier – as well as the increased growth hormone production also alluded to. My logic is that the genetic effects of fasting are developed primarily to enhance survival mechanisms during periods of scarce or erratic food supply. For this reason, when an animal (or person) is faced with potential famine conditions, genetically its survival arsenal is activated. **This means that the senses are sharpened, optimism is increased and energy levels are boosted – in order to bring about a better outcome in the search, fight, or hunt for food.** There are many means of obtaining food under circumstances of increased food scarcity, but most of these methods relate to implementing methods of enhanced competitiveness and ingenuity. Primitive societies of people and animals would probably have had to compete with members of their own species for scarce resources under conditions of famine and this often involved confrontation.

I believe these are the reasons why conditions of food abstinence bring about a heightened sense of alertness and motivation (to go out and better oneself). **It's a genetically programmed survival response.**

To conclude this section, remember that research so far has **proven** that **the only known way to significantly extend mammalian life spans is by controlled starvation - in the absence of malnutrition.** This is a brutal way of paraphrasing "calorie restriction" and - as you will discover when you are fully equipped to take up IF – controlled fasting is nothing close to "brutal" in practice.

The Basics of Intermittent Fasting

There are really only two "basic pillars" of IF, from which all the known regimes can be said to derive. These are:

1. **Alternate Day Fasting (ADF for short).**
2. **Daily Intermittent Fasting using an "Eating Window."**

Both these variants can be said to have been developed off the natural eating patterns familiar to animals that live in the wild (or followed by humans who still live along the same lines as very ancient societies). I will explain the main defining features of these regimes.

Alternate day fasting (ADF) is simply what the name suggests - a scheduled period of fasting, implemented every other day. This normally involves a 24 hour period of regular meals (of the individual's choice and at the preferred meal frequency of that individual), followed by a 24 hour period during which no food and only water - or zero-calorie beverages like black coffee and black/herbal tea - are consumed. The bulk of fasting studies, it must be said, are focused on this particular fasting modality.

Daily IF using "eating windows" is a system of implementing a regular fasting session every day (or most days). The logic used is to restrict all food consumption to what is termed the "eating window." This is a short window period (typically a few hours long) for eating - and it is normally of a fixed time period. The most commonly used time periods for eating windows range between 4 and 6 hours. The determination of duration for eating windows is based around how much weight the individual needs to lose and how active that individual is, physically. If you are very active and only want to lose a little excess fat in order to become very defined and lean, a longer eating window will probably work well. If you are very overweight and not very active, the eating window needs to be dramatically shortened and can even be as brief as just one hour every day (or a single, **well-balanced** meal).

Users of IF need to be aware of the crucial importance of a well-balanced, nutritionally adequate meal. **When eating fewer meals, or consuming fewer calories, the chances of individuals becoming malnourished will statistically increase**. Sometimes a poor diet may be masked when an individual overeats, because the excess food will provide extra nutrient content. Sometimes the excessiveness of consumption is such that even though the nutrient proportions are wrong, underrepresented nutrients are overeaten to the extent that they reach 'adequate' levels.

An example demonstrating the last point made is that of someone consuming only *half* of the required *proportion* of iron in their diet. If this person is over-eating (up to double the healthy calorie requirements for their body) they will not actually be seen to have an iron deficiency - because they will be getting the right quantity of that particular nutrient through overeating. However, as a percentage of total food intake, the

proportion of dietary iron will still only be *half the healthy recommendation*. Should such an individual rationalise food intake (to match the healthy *total quantity recommended)* - suddenly their iron intake will have halved and they will soon become deficient. This example stresses the importance of well-balanced, nutritious food intake when restricting calories.

Remember that fat is lost through fasting **mainly** because fasting serves as a means of restricting calories. **Having said this, if followed correctly (and I will explain how to do so in the next chapter) IF will actually teach you to follow a healthy diet and eat the right things.** This is why it is extremely important to follow IF only when fully informed of **how** to do so.

The "eating window" method of IF is probably more popular because it is slightly more convenient to implement and the fasting periods are somewhat shorter. However, my experience - and the feedback I get from others who are experienced in the different fasting methods - is that the results are virtually the same, whichever method you use – so long as you follow the correct implementation. Having said this, for people who need to lose a great deal of weight, the ADF method is probably easier to enforce **correctly** because there is less likelihood of binge eating. Binge eating can derail an IF regime, which is another reason to only take up the practice when fully informed. **The phasing of foods taken whenever the fast is broken will play a huge role in how successful fasting is** and it is essential that IF users learn how to do this (again, I will outline how this is done in the next chapter).

There are numerous variations of both these basic IF methods, which I will cover in the next chapter.

Different Fasting Regimes

Remember that all fasting must be supported by regular, high, water consumption - throughout the fasting/abstinence period. This is the key to keeping hunger sensations away and keeping the digestive system 'cleansed.' This chapter will cover the various IF methodologies and their offshoots and will also explain **how** to implement them **effectively and conveniently**. **Convenience** of a lifestyle modification is **as important** as **effectiveness**.

My advice is that you read through all the different options carefully and **select one option which you think will best suit your personal circumstances**. Stick to that single methodology for at least 3 months before you can make an objective evaluation of its efficacy. If you have lost an average of about 2 pounds per week **over the 2nd and 3rd months** of the program then you will have derived the maximum expected results for that period and you should probably stick with the program and continue to monitor progress at 3 month intervals - until you reach your ideal bodyweight.

If you have not derived a satisfactory fat burning effect after 3 months you may need to alter the program to better suit your objectives, or choose a more effective (or more convenient) variation of IF. However, **these evaluations are only valid if you have followed the chosen program correctly over the full 3 month period**. You need to be totally honest with yourself during this process and decide if you have genuinely followed a calorie restriction program - or if you have half-heartedly gone about it.

Before we go into the details of the different IF programs it is important to note that **fasting for weight loss must be done in a goal-oriented environment**. This means that you must know **before** you take up an IF regime **what** you are trying to achieve and **how** it can be **objectively** measured. Weight loss goals should not be decided ignorantly and a formula of some sort is required to do this.

People who are not very active, physically - and who do little or no exercise - can use the standard weight-to-height ratio Body Mass Index (BMI) charts as a guide to an ideal healthy weight. But I prefer **a more objective goal** is used, such as the measurement of actual body fat percentage. Not everyone has easy and reliable access to such monitoring so **the next best thing is to use body weight measurements**. Bert Herring, in his intermittent fasting book called "The Fast-5 Diet," recommends a good method for setting weight loss goals using a **calculation of ideal body weight, based on your height and build**. I will outline his recommendations below:

- For women - start with 100 pounds for 5 feet tall and add 5 pounds for every inch above 5 feet tall. Similarly, for men - begin with 106 pounds for 5 feet tall and add 6 pounds for every inch above 5 feet tall.

- Add an extra 10% to the final calculated figure for a large frame, or deduct a further 10% for a small frame (for both men and women).
- It's important not to get misled by this "large frame" and "small frame" terminology. A lot of people use these terms to cover up or excuse improper body weight. "Large frame" does not refer to your weight and that "big boned" phrase is more often misused than used to accurately describe one's true structure.
- There is an objective way to make these determinations and Herring gives a good option. He states that one should **measure wrist circumference to determine frame type**. He recommends cutting a strip of paper at least 8 inches long. Wrap it around your wrist (at the narrowest section, I'd suggest) and mark the circumference on the paper strip. Use that measurement to compare to specified criteria, which will be explained shortly.
- Basically, if you are female and under 5'2" - you have a small frame if your wrist measures less than 5.5" and a large frame if it measures over 5.75". Medium would be 5.5"-5.75"
- For women up to 5'5" tall - under 6" wrist circumference indicates a small frame and over 6.25" a large frame. Medium is from 6.0"-6.25".
- For women over 5'5" tall - a small frame would have a wrist measurement of less than 6.25" and a large frame over 6.5". A medium frame would range from 6.25"-6.5" in wrist circumference.
- For men the measurements are a wrist circumference less than 6.5" for small frames and over 7.5" for large frames. A medium frame ranges from 6.5"-7.5" in wrist circumference.

I hope you'll make use of Dr Herring's chart – or similar - before setting out on a weight loss journey. However, be wary of the fact that very muscular athletic physiques may not conform to any of the formulae outlined above and some intuition will be required to decide when enough weight has been lost. **The best system to use in such instances is accurate body fat monitoring**. If you cannot do this, you are forced to rely on an **objective visual assessment** of muscle definition. Get someone whom you can really rely on to give this assessment - or use clear photographs and assess yourself. **The mirror is not a good option for visual self-assessment.**

I will now begin my outline of different IF regimens by covering the two "basic pillars" of IF (outlined earlier) and then extending my coverage to the other forms of IF which have been (or can be) derived from the two basic 'parent' regimes. I have experimented with the routines to be described in order to get more personal feedback on their practicalities over a reasonable course of time.

ADF

The modality of alternate day fasting is that **fasts are carried out at 24 hour intervals**. To be fair, one can vary that length of time slightly and mark the fasts using actual days (such as Tuesday, Thursday, Friday and Sunday, etc). In fact, using actual calendar days – instead of 24 hour periods – is probably a more 'natural' way of doing this because calendar days are what the body tends to recognise in terms of circadian rhythm. If you followed a calendar-day-based ADF routine your fasts would actually be for more like 32 hours each time - unless you were to get up at night to eat (which is quite unnecessary). However, if you want to time exactly 24 hours each time you fast under this regimen, that should be absolutely fine too and will still allow you to be able to eat every day (if you schedule the start and end times in such a way that they correspond with traditional mealtimes).

In order to take up ADF there are a variety of introductions you can use, based on your personal outlook and physiological/psychological response.

The **simplest** way to commence is to simply start following the regime, with no real breaking-in period. I don't think it's necessarily the **best** way to start and, indeed, it may not even be necessary. However, simple is sometimes best - for some. I've done this "immediate start" routine and it's worked fine for me in the past, but I will not assume this is necessarily the case for everyone.

My observation, anecdotally, is that **the more obese an individual is, the harder it is to totally abstain from eating**. There is a good scientific explanation for this, linked to the enzyme secretions occurring in the adipose (fat) tissues. Adipose tissues secrete a number of hormones and enzymes (many of which are still undocumented) and it is strongly believed that some of these hormones influence appetite and weight stabilisation (as well as issues such as metabolic syndrome and tendency towards diabetes and cardiovascular disease). This is why it becomes very difficult to change your weight (upwards or downwards) when it has been stable for a long time. You literally **get used to the new bodyweight** (physiologically speaking) once it has been stable for a long enough period and it becomes pre-set, much like a thermostat. Hormones and enzymes mediate this response.

For these very reasons, it is imperative that obese individuals make the effort, as difficult as it may be, to break this "hold" that adipose tissue has over their appetite and their relationship with food. **Abstinence is probably the most effective method of breaking chemically mediated "addictions"** and food addiction is real – as I've just explained. Rather than try to regulate eating by "drip feeding" yourself with smaller portions of food more regularly, you'd do well to **totally abstain**. This is where IF comes into it's own. You would not ask a drug addict or an alcoholic to simply "cut down." That is impractical. **Abstinence is the key**. The easiest way for us to regulate eating is to moderately eat the foods of our choice (until fully satiated) during permitted periods – and then to abstain at all other times when we should not be eating. **It's really that simple**.

Regulating small food portions to restrict calories requires tremendous willpower when done over long periods of time and although it is not impossible (a small minority do this very successfully, for long periods), most people cannot seem to do it and have failed (as evidenced by the obesity crisis now firmly established in all societies where food is easily accessed and it is culturally "normal" to eat regularly throughout the day). Not all societies eat liberally - all day long – and this is evidenced by very ancient societies, such as the South American Indians and African "Bushmen" - where obesity is non-existent and people only have one main daily meal (and don't always eat every day).

The longest-living societies in the world all have one thing in common, **they follow near vegetarian diets - with such low calories that they would be considered "starvation diets" by Western standards** - and they get a great deal of **physical exercise** through daily, survival-related chores (such as agriculture, building and hunting). They also follow a lifestyle characterised by **less frequent meals**. I am not suggesting for a moment that you take up a minimalist lifestyle (similar to a rural mountain villager's) but the concepts for good health through lifestyle still should (and can) hold true in a modernised version of the "long-life" diet - such as IF.

Using the every other day (ADF) method is recommended for those who have a lot of weight to lose, because the total weekly calorie restriction (fasting time) is considerable. Also, because there is time for frequent meals on the 'eating days,' it's probably easier to adhere to reasonable eating practices than when you only eat one meal a day. Whichever method of fasting you choose must, first and foremost, be **practical. The most successful weight loss solution is the one that is the most practical**.

The main challenge with ADF, over the long term, is the **regularity** of the lengthy fasting periods. During a period of purposeful weight loss, this sacrifice is reasonable. But **after weight loss goals have been met** there will be a need to scale up the amount of food eaten on the 'eating days' in order to balance the calorie intake and achieve **calorie neutrality**. However, the challenge of alternate day fasting (under conditions during which no weight loss is being sought) may become a burden - especially because **the fasting periods for ADF are the longest ones recommended in standard IF protocols**.

There is a way around this hurdle using the two options to be outlined below:

1. **Instead of total abstinence on the fasting days** in an ADF protocol you can either consume a calorie restricted diet (with only about 40% of your normal daily calorie requirements consumed) or follow a diet based on low calorie, fresh, raw fruits (**as listed in the table to be outlined later in this chapter**). Even if you chose to follow the low calorie fruit option you must still place a **limit on total** calories consumed on the low calorie days (a good guide is about **10 portions** of fresh fruit and vegetables - in total - throughout the low calorie day). The 10 fresh fruit portions can be eaten in just 2 or 3 distinct meals (at traditional mealtimes) or they can be eaten randomly – or evenly – across the 24 hour period. **Do what's most convenient for you**.
2. The second option is based on the fact that it's been found that **many people can actually meet their weight loss goals by fasting just twice - or even once - weekly** (for 24 hours each time). This leads to a variation of ADF where fasting is carried out every 2, 3 - or even 5 -

days. **You can simply reduce the number of fasting days each week if you have reached your weight loss target**. A popularly promoted blueprint for doing this is the Eat Stop Eat Program (popularised by a Canadian nutritionist named Brad Pilon). I've read a lot of Brad's work now - and have also done some collaboration with him for my magazine column - and I can confirm he is among the most learned authorities on IF in the world today. Having said this, for commercial reasons, Brad is probably restricted to promoting just one method of fasting (Eat Stop Eat) and, thus, will only ever address queries along those lines (or recommend solutions around his program alone). I don't think that's a weakness, though – because, **if adhered to correctly, all rational IF methodologies will work for all people** (and Eat Stop Eat is a rational fasting method). That's a massive, sweeping generalisation and I don't make it without due consideration for what I have said. But I believe it is **the truth - calorie restriction will always effect fat loss** (if carried out correctly). Pilon doesn't say much about what to eat - or how to eat - during the 'normal' eating days, when using his program, but I think most people who have the diligence and discipline to take up this new way of eating will be rational enough to realise that **what** you eat (on "eating days") - and **how much** - actually counts.

Eat moderately/conservatively on all eating days, when following ADF, but **eat foods that you like,** so that you don't develop harmful cravings – and eat enough to stop you from feeling hungry throughout the eating day. **All foods, in moderation, are okay during eating windows and/or eating days.** Fasting allows periods of discipline to be interspersed with periods of laxity. **Without some regular measure of 'indulgence,' long term dietary discipline is very difficult for the majority of people to maintain**. Even the fittest and trimmest of us often alternate between periods of leanness and periods of relative obesity. This is common among top athletes, boxers and bodybuilders - and proves the rule applies even for the very best at weight management (and also to those who manipulate their weight for a living). **Periods of discipline must be interspersed with periods of laxity** – ignore this warning at your peril (it is the basis of IF philosophy).

Structuring an Eating Window for ADF or other IF regimes:

On eating days, when following ADF of any variety, you are generally permitted to eat as you like, with some moderation. So that can be 2, 3, 4 or even 5 meals – as you see fit. However, the aim is to keep the eating on the eating days as close to normal as possible (normal being what you eat when not using IF, with considerations for healthy nutrition and reasonable portions).

I usually suggest eating **only low calorie FRESH fruits & vegetables** during most of the day **(outside of the main eating window of that day) - and to support this with regular water consumption**. Eating windows **can** still be used for ADF - **if you eat low calorie fruits during the "fasting" period of the day.** Set aside about 3-5 hours for the eating window each eating day -

during which a balanced diet of your choice is followed, in quantities which suit you. For ADF you can extend that window period to up to 8 hours total duration, if that works for you (on the eating day, of course). You can follow this "eating window" method of eating during ADF regimes, **even though many would consider it to be a stand-alone form of IF on its own** (thus, **2 methods of IF can be followed simultaneously when practicing ADF**).

A list of good low calorie fruits is shown below:

Fruit/Vegetable	Amount (Portion)	Calories
Apple	1	47
Apricot	1	12
Banana	1	95
Cherry	1	2
Clementine	1	22
Fruit salad	1 portion	84
Grapefruit	1	100
Grapes	1	3
Kiwi	1	30
Mango	1	86
Melon (Cantaloupe) (Honeydew)	1 slice 1 slice	30 56
Nectarine	1	60
Orange	1	60
Peach	1	50
Pear	1	53
Pineapple	1 ring	20
Plum	1	20
Prickly pear	1	50
Satsuma	1	25
Strawberries	1	5
Watermelon	1 slice	60

Use your preferred FRESH, raw fruits and vegetables - as long as you keep portion sizes below 100 calories during actual fasting periods - and try to restrict yourself to 5 portions during the bulk of the day, during fasting periods (you can have more during the actual eating window, if

you want). 5-9 daily fruit and vegetable portions are recommended by nutritional experts and I think this is a reasonable practice to follow when using IF (for the low calorie/fasting day). I personally prefer to eat mainly apples, pears, nectarines and bananas if I do eat during fasting periods (outside my eating windows). I suggest that you feel free to use the fresh, raw fruits or vegetables which suit you best (in restricted quantities, as suggested).

In the actual eating window **all fresh fruits** (in reasonable quantities) are okay to eat **- so long as they don't fill you up to the point where you can't eat a complete, fully-balanced and nutritional meal within the scheduled eating window period**. You should generally break the fast (commence the eating window period) by eating low calorie fruits and vegetables – to avoid the risk of binge eating and to avoid insulin spikes (which are usually followed by an energy crash - or a period of fatigue and sluggishness).

So, in short, you can basically eat as much as you comfortably can take in of 'ordinary food' during the actual eating window period. **The meal must cover your minimum nutritional requirements** and you should only eat until comfortably full during eating windows. **You should not feel hungry at the end of an eating window,** but you need to learn to distinguish between "hunger" and the psychological desire to keep eating needlessly (a problem most overweight people will have, which is part of the phenomenon commonly termed as "comfort eating"). **One very full stomach per day will never make a person obese** – just ensure you eat nutritionally valid food to avoid potential deficiencies and to prevent hunger in the next day's low intake phase - and be strict in your calorie restriction by observing disciplined fasting periods.

A good way to avoid comfort eating during eating windows is to plan what you are going to eat in advance and to include as many different foods and food types in that meal as you can. However, because you will probably have to **eat all your food at one sitting**, ensure the portions are small enough for you to eat everything **comfortably**. By **eating everything in one sitting you are less likely to overeat** (with regard to total, daily caloric intake) because your appetite will be fully satisfied. **I recommend this approach to all eating windows for most IF protocols. Eat all your food for the eating window period at one sitting, whenever possible, in order to restrict calories to the capacity of just one full stomach each day.**

The 'window period' really refers to when you can start and when you must finish your eating, but it **does not stipulate constant eating for the full duration – unless metabolic demands drive this** (which can genuinely happen for very active athletes who train heavily). If you are not a heavy training athlete you need to be careful about how much eating you permit in eating windows.

A good way of determining when you've had enough is suggested by Ori Hofmekler in his IF book called "The Warrior Diet". He says "stop eating when reasonably full and take a 20 minute break to determine if you are still genuinely hungry." It takes 20 minutes for hunger signals to stop transmitting - even if you are full - another reason to **always eat slowly**.

He also suggests eating the foods with the mildest tastes first. This is one of the most important rules for breaking bingeing habits and I am a strong believer in this. I also believe it is best to **break all fasts with low calorie FRESH fruits** (see the list provided earlier).

Eat as much low calorie fresh fruit as it takes to lose the 'bingeing feeling' when you first open your eating window, each day. The same applies for the first meal on an eating day when following ADF without the use of eating windows. After this, eat your fully balanced meal. **If still hungry after a normal-sized plate of food, you can eat yet more fruit** (even not-so-low-calorie fruits, because most fruits and vegetables are healthy).

Hofmekler suggests eating the highest calorie and highest GI foods **last in the eating window**. He also suggests eating whatever you consider to be the best tasting foods last. This approach works well if you can make it practical. Don't get too caught up in the stipulations and minor details of phasing foods - keep it practical and do what you need to do to ensure you don't binge during the eating window. Eat the healthiest, lowest calorie and **lowest GI** foods first (and in bulk) - or you will negate the calorie restriction aspect of IF (which is required to burn off excess fat).

"Glycemic Index" (GI) refers to the levels of fast-releasing sugars in foods. High GI indicates more 'sugary' carbohydrates (which release quickly and cause a sudden insulin overproduction, in order to clear the bloodstream of the excess sugar) and low GI refers to more complex, slow-releasing carbohydrates (which encourage a healthy insulin production profile, with lower insulin secretions overall). Good health is a result of keeping the GI low because that leads to lower insulin production **and increased growth hormone production** – meaning a less fat (leaner), more muscular body (growth hormone promotes muscular development).

There are two advantages to using fruits and very mild tasting, low calorie foods to break and control fasts. Firstly, they prevent binge eating (I know of nobody who binges on fresh fruits & vegetables - and simultaneously has a weight problem). Secondly, eating this way stops you feeling hungry during the fasting period which follows - and over the next day (this is **probably the most important outcome** because it **teaches and enforces good eating habits** and overall portion control). Eating this way also suggests that you are 'smoothing out' your blood glucose profile (because it is erratic insulin production from over-consumption of high GI/glycemic index meals that leads to poor appetite control and erratic energy levels).

Also be aware of the fact that **the slimmer you become using this method the better your appetite-moderation/control will become,** because the unhealthy hormonal production caused by excessive fat reserves is improved/reduced as the bulk/quantity of fat reduces. As previously explained, being fat actually causes a hormonal profile that encourages hunger signals,

29

which is why obese people have such difficulty controlling their eating and this is part of what is commonly called the "metabolic syndrome" or "Syndrome X." Yes, **being fat does encourage you to become fatter** - from a purely biochemical and physiological perspective.

Daily IF using Eating Windows

Now that we've looked at pure ADF, it's pertinent to look at the other founding pillar of IF - **regular daily fasting**. This involves a set fasting period each day, with a fixed eating window of typically 3-6 hours. **4 or 5 hours for eating window periods appear to work best for most people.** Some users of IF believe women should use larger eating windows than men - and that women **should not** aim to reduce total body fat percentage to the same extent as men. I believe there is some validity to this outlook but it is not of great physiological significance.

From a purely social perspective, most women do not aim to be as lean and rugged in appearance as many men do, so a body fat percentage of 10-15% may suit many women well (and will give the sort of body toning results most women prefer). Women will often begin to look very wiry once they get to around 10% body fat. By using a longer eating window period - and perhaps 'grazing' a bit more across the duration of this window period - it is easy to limit fat loss (once your body fat is getting quite low). **But longer eating windows should only be used when body fat is already quite low – and not at the beginning of a weight loss program.** The length of eating window is the best way to move between active weight loss and general maintenance of ideal weight. As mentioned, only do so when you are at around your ideal goal bodyweight.

As mentioned earlier, **follow the rules for breaking the fast using the least flavoured and/or lowest calorie foods** (ideally fresh, low calorie fruits). Also, use the window period as a guide to cover when all your main eating activity should take place. Don't feel obliged to 'graze' throughout the window period. **Aim for just one main meal** - even if it is a 3 course meal. **This way, it is virtually impossible to overeat because stomach capacity becomes a limiting factor.** Plan your meals in advance - so that you know what you are going to eat (and in which order). **Sweets (if eaten) should be last in the eating window** and you must not feel that they are essential eating - unless you still crave them after eating everything else. **Use fruits to bulk up meals and try to eat a main meal of the same size as you would if you were regularly eating all through the day.**

If you exercise (which, ideally all people should) then try to time exercise sessions for within one hour on either side of your main meal. If your schedule makes this impossible, just eat some low calorie fresh fruit **before and after** exercising and this will tide you over until the main meal (even if done in the morning during the fasting period, when the eating window is set for the evening). **As a rule, do not consume more than 5 portions of FRESH fruit and vegetables during the fasting period - and it will still meet the physiological criteria of being a genuine fast**.

If you are new to this, a good way to "break yourself in" is to either skip your breakfast completely - and reduce to just 2 meals a day – before eventually reducing to just one eating window period for each day. Or you can set breakfast back by an hour – every consecutive day, until it merges with lunchtime - and continue the process until lunchtime merges with the eating window (traditional dinner time). **Eating windows can be any time of day** that suits you. Let convenience – and the times you exercise - be the main determinants of when your eating window is.

Eat whatever decent foods you like in the actual eating window, but try to adhere to the suggested sequencing rules outlined earlier (e.g. start your eating with fresh fruits). Don't feel bad about having breakfast cereal after 'supper' if you strongly feel like doing so (I do this almost daily to boost carbohydrate intake). But keep high calorie, so-called "highly processed foods" to the end of the eating window - so that your appetite is small and your consumption of these foods is, thus, kept low (this would include bread, cereals, deserts and chocolates, etc).

Please Note:

These sequencing rules are still important - even if you don't tend to binge - because they prevent hunger pangs the next day (in the fasting period).

Be prepared, when fasting regularly using the daily (or almost daily) method that once your metabolism is fully adjusted (after about a month of using the practice) you may find yourself becoming **more sensitive to cold weather – especially during the actual fasting periods**. Many people feel colder than normal once the fasting metabolism becomes fully developed (using the daily fasting method). It's to be expected – even if you follow the version whereby you eat 5 portions of fruit and vegetables during the eating window - and is nothing to worry about. Dress warmly on cold days.

Rules for the Fasting Period of the day:

During fasts, **consume mainly water**. Zero-calorie diet drinks can occasionally be taken, but in minimal quantities. This recommendation is made for 2 reasons. Firstly, diet drinks **may** promote a significant insulin response, as some research suggests, which invalidates genuine fasting. This violates the physiological fasting criteria of low insulin secretion and encourages hunger pangs, energy fluctuations and often causes general psychological discomfort. Secondly, these drinks are not healthy and high consumption of them over many months and years may lead to health problems in later life. This is not proven directly but is highly likely, considering how unnatural the constituents of these drinks are. Remember – **moderation** for everything you eat. Not much is totally off bounds, in terms of foods, but some things need considerable restriction for health to be maintained.

Starting fasts can be done in a number of ways under the daily fasting method. Dr Bert Herring's Fast-5 program gives a number of very practical solutions for starting a fasting regime of this sort and I highly recommend it as one of the best books available on daily fasting, using a short eating window. The simplest method, as always, is to commence outright ("cold turkey, as Herring refers to it).

I actually recommend "cold turkey" as the best way to start - with a caveat. **Always carry a stash of fresh fruit with you when you are new to this methodology**. If you begin to feel uncomfortable - or feel any unusual sensations - don't feel bad about eating an apple or two, or even a full complement of 5 whole portions of fresh fruit in one sitting. You will discover later in this chapter that **I am a huge advocate of using the recommended 5 daily portions of fresh fruit and vegetables as a key part of intermittent fasting**, either to break fasts and commence an eating window, or to tide you over during the actual fasting period (if you are having very bad hunger pangs).

Having used IF for a long time now, at the time of going to print I've **never** had problems with significant hunger spells during fasts and have never failed to complete a scheduled fast. IF is not hard to do for me. But I will not make the sweeping assumption that this will be the case for everyone - at the beginning. However, after a few months of trial and adjustment - and by using a variety of different IF alternatives, **the practice becomes very easy for everyone – eventually**. A little patience may be required by some, but it's worth the perseverance. As explained earlier, especially the overweight may initially struggle with hunger pangs, due to excessive hormonal secretions caused by having larger quantities of body fat. But this should pass.

I strongly believe that part-time fasting is the best way to start using IF because it allows successful 'cold turkey' commencement - which leads to quicker adaptation and lifestyle change. To do this, begin IF just one day a week; then add on another **non-consecutive** day (after a month, or so, of trialling the single day fasts) and continue adding additional fasting days, weekly - from then onwards - until most of your week uses the IF methodology. **You may never need to go to full-time daily fasting** (but the more overweight, or those after faster results, will find full-time fasting suits their needs better). I think fasting on most days will work for most people - as a long term lifestyle change. Daily fasting, without breaks, may lead to increased gorging during the eating windows - or may lead to boredom with the routine for many individuals.

You can vary the routine by adding modified fasts, which involve the consumption of 5 portions of raw, low calorie fruits or vegetables during the fasting period. This is a great method for introducing variety to a daily fasting routine - without diminishing its effectiveness - and is my preferred fasting method.

When you have reached your pre-determined ideal weight I think **part-time fasting regimes** - or regimes which don't involve daily periods of abstinence - are actually **more suitable, for weight maintenance purposes. The routine need not be very rigid, when you are at a good bodyweight.** This way, it can become a full-time, long term lifestyle choice and long term health and weight maintenance can be secured. The popular Eat Stop Eat program uses this philosophy - and anecdotal observations suggest it works well for most people who try it. It is a form of ADF and I personally prefer daily fasting to ADF, but they are equally effective and many people prefer ADF. See which one suits you by trying both methods (over different time periods), for variety.

Having looked at the two main methods of IF, I will now outline hybrids and variations/combinations which can be used to make these methods more adaptable, to better suit all tastes and circumstances. Please note at this point that you should resist the urge to constantly "hybridise" methods as a way of making fasting easier, because most of these methods can only be said to have been implemented effectively if followed for at least a week at a time - and I strongly believe people new to IF should **stick to just one method for a minimum of 3 months before even considering tweaking it.**

- Also, **expect to lose no more than 2 pounds a week – on average.**
- **The first month of IF should not see much weight loss – if any at all.**
- **Expect it to take up to 6 months before IF becomes a completely normal way of eating for you (to the extent that you actually will resist following your previous eating methods).**
- **If a particular method works well for you, stick with it as long as you are getting results. Remember, you can only lose 2 pounds a week, at best, so if you are 100 pounds overweight it will take a year to reach ideal weight and to show full muscle definition.**
- **If you begin an exercise program at the same time as a weight loss program, you must face the possibility of changing your end goals. Exercise may increase your muscle mass so that even when losing fat your weight does not decrease correspondingly. But don't use this concept to fool yourself - *you cannot gain muscle mass at nearly the same rate as you can lose fat.* In real terms, a 10% increase in target minimum weight is probably practical in most cases where *significant* exercise is introduced at the same time as weight loss measures.**
- **Don't be surprised if you become more sensitive to cold weather after a few months of fasting. This is an indication that your body has learned to run almost entirely on free fatty acids during fasting periods (and this type of metabolism doesn't liberate as much heat as glucose metabolism - much like diesel motors run at lower temperatures than more explosive petrol engines, if such an analogy helps).**

Now it's time for our look at the varieties of IF routines available.

Modified ADF:

You can modify an ADF regime in a number of ways.

- So, instead of total abstinence on the "fasting" day, you can consume meals of just fresh fruit and vegetables on that day instead. If total calories are restricted to about 40% of what you should normally be eating on a "normal" day, this will still count as ADF and should be almost equally effective (when compared to total abstinence). However, I am a big believer in observing some sort of regular "genuine fasting" period, where 'true abstinence' is observed. So I recommend that **if you choose this option, you should still try to observe at least one "genuine" abstinence fast each week**.

- Another modified ADF routine will be to observe a "normal" eating day - followed by a day of intermittent fasting (whereby you observe a fasting period with a short eating window - on alternating days). **This is a direct hybrid between the two main fasting methods**.

- **Eat Stop Eat** is yet another version of modified ADF, as promoted by Brad Pilon, and serves as a way of following ADF with fewer fasting days/more eating days between fasts. He suggests just 2 non-consecutive fasting days each week (24 hours at a time), until you minimise your weight. You can then reduce to one fasting day each week, to maintain muscle definition and weight loss.

- Similar to Eat Stop Eat is modified ADF routine in which you fast every 2 days, rather than every other day. **This would work also as an introduction to ADF – or as a permanent methodology for people who are not overweight but still want to improve their muscle definition by losing a little fat.**

- The possibility exists to modify the rules of the latter-mentioned fasting method and fast for 2 consecutive days, followed by 2 days of normal eating – and so on. I have never tried this personally, but the theoretical protocol does exist in the literature and in the studies I have read. **I suspect it is not very practical for the majority of people and I only mention it for academic reasons**. My feeling is that fasting for too long (much longer than 24 hours) may harm protein sparing and lead either to muscle degradation or to suppression of muscular development in individuals trying to build up strength and muscularity.

- A possible way of doing a consecutive days (48 hour) fast could involve using the modified fasting strategy alluded to earlier in this handbook, consuming 5-10 portions of low calorie fruits and vegetables every 24 hour period during the fast. Scientifically speaking, there is no reason why this should not work - if the particular scheduling appeals to you.

There are also a number of permutations possible for the **daily method of IF using a short eating window**. They are outlined below:

- **You can choose to consume up to 5 portions of fresh, raw fruits and vegetables during the fasting period – almost every day**. I would envisage people using this method for **maintenance,** when minimum target weight has been attained; and it is one of my personal favourites - **although I still suggest one or two days where a genuine abstinence is observed during the fasting period**. For those who are not particularly overweight it can be **a good way to start IF (also useful for those who find total abstinence difficult at the outset).** You will probably find, using this method, that eventually you will not feel any hunger and will need to will yourself to consume the fruits during fasting periods (which is what I usually experience). If this is the case, you can use genuine fasts on some days and fruit fasts on others. Just ensure you do at least one or two genuine fasts every week.

You can commence this method in a number of ways:

1. The fruits can be split up into a distinct breakfast and lunch.
2. They can be eaten in just one meal.
3. They can be randomly consumed across the 19-21 hour fasting period of the day.

Always break the fast (i.e. open the eating window) using fresh fruits - even if you consume 5 fruit portions during the fasting period itself. I prefer to have the fruits in just one meal, at lunchtime. There are 3 reasons for this. Firstly, it allows a genuine 15 hour fast, with some complete abstinence, every day. Secondly, it allows me to fit into the social eating structures prevalent in most of society (because lunch and supper are usually the most communal, shared meals). And lastly, eating at breakfast time primes an insulin response (albeit a small one) early in the day - which actually makes you more susceptible to hunger pangs during the rest of the fasting period for that day. **It's easier not to eat at all - during fasts - than to eat just a little at a time.**

- **Random daily fasting** can be performed by alternating between "genuine" fasts - with total abstinence - and random days of "fruit fasting". This is good for variety **when you are at minimum body fat**. This is also a good way of being able to continue with IF for indefinite periods.
- Earlier in this handbook I mentioned **The Warrior Diet,** written by Ori Hofmekler. He brands it as an IF regime for athletes and there are a number of well-known international athletes who are known to follow his routine. As an avid IF user I must admit I only became more fully acquainted with Ori's work quite recently, during a collaboration for my magazine column - despite the relative international popularity of The Warrior Diet. Having read the book now I must say it was a decent read, in my opinion - but not as concise and engaging as I would have hoped - and it dwelt heavily on the promotion of a myriad of food

supplements. For this reason, some IF beginners could possibly find the information confusing - or even overwhelming. For seasoned users of IF, however, I think it would probably make a very good and relatively entertaining read. A summary of my take on this mode of IF would be as follows:

I think the general recommendations to be drawn from The Warrior Diet - between all the information on various food supplements and the numerous rules about which foods to eat, or not to eat - is that **Ori promotes very healthy, organic, and low-sugar eating, along the lines of a modified IF protocol (much like my '5 a day' fruit preference).** I think The Warrior Diet is genuinely a modified IF protocol (in much the same way as the modified ADF variations outlined earlier in this handbook which rely on just fruits or vegetables on low calorie 'fasting' days).

Ori suggests a low calorie, low GI, vegetarian/vegan diet during the first 20 hours of each day – called the "under-eating" or "fasting" phase of the diet – followed by a 4 hour eating window, which he refers to as the "overeating" phase (during which you eat to full satiety).

That's the Warrior Diet in a nutshell. Protein shakes, containing fast-assimilating whey protein, are also promoted during the "fasting" or "under-eating" phase of this diet and I believe this diet is actually a good compromise between traditional IF and the multiple meal, low calorie, "ultra-clean" diets already popular in bodybuilding and physical culture. It certainly fits in well with my preferred "off season" routine of raw fruits all day (in the "fasting period" before the eating window) and I have no doubt it's a great way for heavy training athletes and bodybuilders to use an IF model with somewhat less restriction of calories.

In defence of the "picky eating" encouraged in The Warrior Diet, there is no reason why "ultra clean" eating cannot be a part of an IF regime (but it must be said that the majority of IF devotees are often those who defaulted to the method primarily because they found it difficult to be "picky" and exact about everything they ate – and about when to eat it). IF is about following a few very basic rules and eating relatively flexibly – using fasting periods to regulate total potential food intake and to balance out 'loose' eating habits during eating windows or eating days. I strongly suggest that IF users avoid overly unhealthy foods (as Ori suggests) wherever possible - and focus mainly on **overall calorie restriction** by using periods of phased eating, sandwiched between periods of phased abstinence.

There is value in both the calorie restriction and in the periods of abstinence themselves. Traditional low calorie diets can offer the same CR benefits as IF, if calories are effectively reduced – as competitive bodybuilders have demonstrated very well over the years - but they cannot offer the **genetic advantages** of a regular period of total abstinence.

I am sometimes asked if IF truly works for bodybuilders - and I find that a difficult question to answer in a totally scientific way.

36

To summarise, **I do believe IF works for pure bodybuilders**. However, there are not many credible real-life examples to offer as proof. You may question why I hold my particular beliefs - if that is the case (regarding proof and real-life examples)? Really, I base it on my own experiences and observations - of both myself and other IF users I know of. I have not seen any reduction in muscularity myself, since I started using IF. Quite the opposite, actually. And this seems to commonly be the case with users of IF. The problem here is that I am **not** a bodybuilder - and the type of individual who is a genuine bodybuilder (in the same cast as the huge guys we see in the magazines) is unlikely to ever veer towards trying something different or new for achieving muscle definition.

This sounds like a mean generalisation when I state it that way, but I do not mean it maliciously. **The culture in bodybuilding is almost an exact opposite/mirror image of that seen in anorexics – and is similarly extreme**. There is a high prevalence of **body dimorphic perception** present in bodybuilding culture - so that athletes never see themselves in their true light. They always see themselves as being smaller and less-developed than they actually are and the literature (promoted by supplement manufacturers and drug peddlers, really) implies that muscle mass can be lost very easily by just doing small things differently to the blueprint they recommend.

In other words, the mainstream approach to bodybuilding (because it is an insular sport, promoted by a small clique of people with a commercial interest in selling supplements), is that '**a shotgun is used to shoot a tiny mouse**.' **The approach promoted (in order to brainwash bodybuilders into reliance on supplements) is that more is better**. More of everything – more training, more eating, more sleeping, more supplements - and more drugs. As I just said, **it does work** – because nothing is left to chance. Yes, **the shotgun-type approach will work**. But it need not be that way, if training and dieting is done with high levels of precision and understanding.

The smart (and modern) athlete seeks to know - and understand - *why* things are done; and puts every hypothesis to test. A modern athlete **questions everything** and **treats time with value**. Using that approach, **it quickly becomes evident that you can get to your maximum genetic potential on literally half the things the magazines try to convince you are necessary to get there** – if you **pressure test every single thing you do** - so as to reduce activities to only those which are maximally effective and minimally time-consuming.

Your muscles will not atrophy just because you miss one of your 3-hourly protein shakes or supplement tablets (which is the suggestion given by the magazines). **The human body is resistant to change** and does not make sudden changes based on minor variations in routine over the short term. The truth is, those supplements make little difference to people who are not malnourished and **there is no need for ridiculously high protein intake to build big muscles**. The major factor in the development of **all** professional bodybuilders' physiques is the use of performance-enhancing steroid-type drugs, coupled with intense physical training.

Supplements have little to do with it - although users of such steroids can actually process unnatural amounts of food, which will incorporate into muscle tissues – something **impossible for drug free athletes**. So whichever way you view this topic - from a purely scientific perspective, **the supplements are not the deciding factor. The key deciding factors in professional bodybuilding are the drugs and the intense training.** Supplements, in these cases, allow more convenient ingestion of high quantities of calories. **Such high numbers of calories are meaningless in the absence of drugs** - except for the most extreme cases of **professional** athletes who train very long and very hard, such as **professional** runners.

It is only through the use of drugs that a human body can meaningfully synthesize the amounts of protein and food taken in by professional bodybuilders. If a 'clean' individual attempts to grow his/her muscles though the use of a high calorie diet, driven/enhanced by supplementation, he/she will simply get fat – regardless of how hard he/she tries to exercise. The body cannot utilise food to the extent seen in professional bodybuilding - without considerable 'enhancement' of the hormone pool which drives physical development and fat burning. **Bodybuilding drugs have been reliably proven to curtail people's life spans considerably,** so this is not a venture worth pursuing for any reasonable, health-conscious person.

To validate the points I have just made, I train less than half as much as I did 10 years ago. I also sleep less (although I recommend sleeping for as long as you need to every day) and I train less often than 10 years ago. Despite this, my physique remains virtually identical to how it was in my mid twenties (and considering ten years have passed I think that says a lot). In addition, my martial arts skills have continued to improve yearly - and so have my endurance and my energy levels. **I have done this by training smarter and pressure testing all my fitness activities to prove that they actually are essential for attaining my goals.**

A good example of the point I am illustrating about body building (and cultural resistance to new concepts) is that of a philosophy called high **intensity training – or H.I.T. -** whereby athletes only perform one set of each bodybuilding exercise done in the gym - as opposed to the traditional 3 or 4 sets **– and do not use supplements**. This was said to be unviable for building muscles (in the excessive culture of bodybuilding). Much in the same way as eating 1 meal a day is said to be unviable in the bodybuilding culture today. **This status quo about high intensity training persisted for over 30 years after it was first proven to work, despite many people disproving the fallacy by reaching their best using the high intensity method.** This was because none of the reigning champions used it. So the magazines could sideline the theory despite some fringe bodybuilders - who were almost as good as the champions of the time - actually using HIT.

It was only when the best bodybuilder in the world admitted he only used high intensity training (during the 90's) that the fallacy was exposed. Even then, it was glossed over and played down during his **7 year reign** as champion. But the word was finally out. However, high intensity training is still not acknowledged in mainstream bodybuilding media, despite the large number of prominent athletes who have admitted they train solely in that fashion. So do not assume the status quo is always correct – analyse all the information at your disposal to get to solutions which will suit you uniquely, such as IF.

Back to the issue of IF and bodybuilding - **I am convinced that if an IF user, who wants to become a professional bodybuilder, goes and does the right physical training, for the right period of time - and uses the established drug-taking regimes prevalent in the sport - he/she will still develop to the same extent as if he/she had followed the traditional (shotgun) approach to bodybuilding training**. It has yet to happen, of course - in the same way that it took over 30 years for a bodybuilding champion to emerge using the high intensity training method - **but that does not mean it can't/won't happen**. If numerous drug-free athletes are reaching their physical best while using IF, there is no reason why this logic should not translate to bodybuilding as well. The science says it all.

Remember, many users of IF have reached peak physical condition while following the method – and this includes peak muscle size (for them). I can say the same for myself. Having said this, I cannot see myself - or anyone else - being able to convince a steroid-taking bodybuilder, who aspires to turn professional, into trying IF. They are simply too desperate to take 'risks' of a scientific sort and the culture of excess which has founded the sport is unlikely to allow the opportunity to arise. But **until this is done I do not believe it can be demonstrated that IF will curtail muscular developmental potential for bodybuilders**. **The scientific evidence opposes such a viewpoint.**

One rule of bodybuilding must still be adhered to - if you are to succeed at using IF for bodybuilding. This is that there must be an "off-season" period for "bulking up," followed by a "dieting" period for trimming down and gaining definition. That is the case with the commonly promoted low calorie, multiple meal diets, currently used by bodybuilders - and the same will be true if a bodybuilder were to switch to using IF. **You cannot maximise your muscle building potential under conditions of calorie deficit - or even calorie neutrality. There must be a surplus in overall calories if your muscles are to bulk up to their full potential under conditions of hard strength training.** But seasonally you will still need to trim off the excess fat, in order to prevent fat build-up and a re-setting of your minimum weight (due to enzymes produced by fat tissues).

In summary, you need to lose definition in your physique (by eating more than your body needs to survive) in order to see a peak in muscle size, under heavy training conditions aimed at achieving maximum muscle size. **You need to gain weight (and, thus, get fatter as well) in order to see maximum muscle growth as a result of bodybuilding**. However, the excess weight can be removed again by dieting - without losing too much of the extra muscle gained - and **this cycle is a necessity for building a very muscular body**. But if you are an athlete interested in maintaining good appearance **all year round** that goal is still feasible – as long as you are aware of the fact that a small sacrifice in muscle growth will have to be made.

The facts outlined in the previous paragraph hold true, whether or not you use IF as your weight loss diet of choice.

Exercise

There is a clearly defined role for exercise in weight loss and in IF programs. It is becoming something of a cliché to say this but I mean it in absolute earnest. I actually believe exercise is an essential part of being able to live your full natural lifespan with a reasonable quality of life. **From a purely IF perspective, exercise is essential for activating protein sparing mechanisms to ensure your body doesn't break down muscle proteins as a substitute energy source**.

For people who want to be healthy through intermittent fasting there are 2 aspects of exercise which must be addressed – **"why" and "how."**

Why?

Many of the genetic systems of the human body are designed to suit specific 'environmental' conditions and the full expression of all the genes involved in moderating and regulating lifespan-related issues (these genes are often referred to as the "human genome" - or "genetic program") is dependent on specific conditions prevailing. Already discussed is the significance of intermittent food supplies and regular periods of genuine food abstinence (and overall calorie restriction) on the expression of the human genome. **Also important is the prevalence of regular, intermittent physical activity**.

The scientific reasoning for this is rather complex and I will not claim that I – or anyone else, for that matter – **fully** understand it. There are many gaps in our scientific knowledge – which are constantly being filled in as research progresses – but we will **never** fill them all. So **a leap of faith will always be required when approaching matters relating to *purpose of design***. However, don't let this distract you when searching for the facts.

*The phrase **"use it or lose it"** sums up human genetic expression completely.*

Your genes give you a specified "genetic **potential**." Note emphasis on the word "**potential**." This is because without certain environmental factors prevailing not all genetic potential will be realised. You either use it or you lose it - so to speak. **This is why exercise and calorie restriction/IF are so important.**

- Exercise allows you to fully express your natural genetic physical potential and to live for your full lifespan (as determined by your genes).

- *IF is akin to 'metabolic exercise.'*

Don't forget the last 2 points I've just made, **they are the basis of this lifestyle philosophy** and they **apply to everyone**. The method you use for achieving these goals is yours to choose - but the **facts** remain unchanged.

In this chapter I am simply expressing my beliefs around such issues and how they potentially relate to IF. I believe this philosophy is important for understanding **why** IF is healthy - but remember that whether or not you agree with my particular viewpoints on matters of design, they don't actually change the facts **from which I am working backwards** – so to speak. One of those facts is that **IF has measurable and proven health outcomes** (as well-proven as the claims for any other so-called healthy diet and lifestyle). This fact exists - regardless of our interpretations of **why** it exists. I am simply trying to explain such findings in relation to purpose of design; **I am not trying to prove the findings themselves. The science has already done this for us.**

The "whys" of human and animal design are probably going to present an argument in humanity and philosophy which will never be unanimously resolved and different factions will choose their own interpretations of this aspect of science. That's okay for purposes of this discussion and my hypothesis is based on the universally accepted fact that **animal systems self-regulate themselves using** what are called "**feedback mechanisms**." Feedback Mechanisms behave much like a thermostat (in concept). They keep specific parameters within their functional ranges, so that living systems can stay alive and remain **internally constant** – despite a changing external environment.

For instance, if the normal functional range for blood sugar levels is 4-6 mmols/l this means that the body will 'fight' as hard as it can to maintain these functional parameters. The feedback mechanisms for doing this are 'designed' to **function under specific natural conditions**. These "specific natural conditions" relate to eating a specified amount and type of food, at specified intervals - and specified physical workloads (exercise). For these reasons, it is genetically pre-determined (as a result of 'design') that the feedback mechanisms for blood sugar control will work effectively and efficiently in a certain type of 'environmental setting' involving the factors just listed.

If conditions deviate too far (in either direction) from those expected (and for which the body is designed), the feedback systems will fail. When feedback systems fail to cope with the demands placed on them the organism's health will deteriorate and potential lifespan will be shortened – automatically (because health and lifespan are based on certain ideal parameters being maintained).

Sticking with the blood sugar example above, if you eat too much food (quantity) of a sugary nature (quality), the bloodstream will be 'assaulted' by unhealthy levels of glucose - produced as a result of digesting this food. If your food is too 'sugary' the feedback systems which regulate your internal environment will attempt to lower the sugar overproduction by secreting a high volume of insulin. **If the diet you are consuming today is so far removed from the prevalent diet which existed at the time when the body was initially 'designed' - the feedback systems governing insulin production and metabolism will fail to cope and your sugar levels will not return to the normal range (despite maximal insulin production).**

In the continued striving to achieve the normal blood sugar range by producing more and more insulin **(this striving is something feedback systems are compelled to do - to avoid death)** your feedback system (the pancreas in this example) will actually become exhausted and will begin to deteriorate and malfunction. This leads to the disease condition called *Type 2 diabetes mellitus*. You lose the ability to effectively regulate blood glucose (sugar) levels permanently, as a result of diabetes mellitus (caused by the deterioration of the pancreas and the associated hormonal systems which govern its functioning). **This will lead to deterioration in health and a potentially shortened lifespan - as a direct result.**

This concept applies to all other feedback processes and effectively illustrates the relationship between organism design (genetics) and healthy living (lifestyle factors). We need to do our best to re-create the environmental conditions for which our bodies are design to perform at their best, if we are to reach our true physical and lifespan potential. Thankfully, this is quite easily done, even under very modern conditions. Using IF and following an active lifestyle will take you a long way towards achieving this. **That is why exercise is so important as part of a healthy lifestyle and that is why exercise should be viewed as a normal/essential chore in your routine - much like eating, washing, tooth brushing and drinking water.**

You are genetically designed to function under specific conditions – involving regular exercise and intermittent calorie restriction. Doing otherwise is the equivalent of running a motor on the wrong fuel [in some cases it may run for a while (albeit with a stutter), but it will not last for its specified lifespan and it will eventually break down]. It is your responsibility to make an informed choice about factors which will heavily influence your entire life and this book is intended to help you do so.

How?

Under the intermittent fasting protocols there are a few issues around exercise - which you **must** master. I will list them below:

- **When** to exercise is important. Try to exercise in such a way that your main meal of the day is **within 1 hour of when you exercise**. This could be **before or after** your exercise session, so long as the meal commences within an hour of actual exercise. It's good to have a snack of some sort immediately after exercising (or within 15 minutes of completion). This is not as important when you have eaten your main

43

meal **before** exercising, but it is a good idea if you eat **after** exercising. The body has a window of enhanced processing ability immediately after exercise and this window closes quickly. Failure to exploit this window leads to reduced results from any specified exercise session and delayed recovery (which reduces energy levels in the days after exercising and may also lead to increased susceptibility to opportunistic infections, if you exercise hard).

- **Use a set regularity pattern of exercise - ranging from once weekly to almost every day.** Only very experienced and able individuals can exercise once weekly and still get benefit, because it takes a lot of knowledge and experience to address all the fitness parameters effectively in just one session. Most people will need to exercise 3 times weekly – or more – to get good value out of it. **Regularity of exercise is more important than absolute quality of exercise** (as long as you are exercising correctly). **Incorrect exercise is pointless - and most likely harmful.** Ensure you are **competently** trained in **how** to exercise - don't just 'make it up' as you go along.

- **Exercise all the muscle groups on your body to induce protein sparing across the entire body.** If, say, you only use running for exercise - protein sparing will only really occur in your legs and the rest of your muscles may actually decrease in size, when you are on a weight loss program. **Strength training is better for protein sparing than endurance training.** Do strength work, like lifting weights, if you want to have a defined upper and lower body. If you just do distance running, for instance, you are likely to look like a distance runner - with protein sparing (and hence, muscle definition) just in the legs - and a very slim, undefined upper body.

- **For people new to exercise, an active sport is often a very good idea for getting active.** A word of caution though: **sports are seldom reasonable as a 'complete' and well-rounded exercise program.** Sports use the body unevenly and this is not ideal for general exercise - unless you also follow a conditioning program to balance body strength development, symmetrically.

- **Use a form of exercise which motivates you, because** *regularity* **over the long term is much more important than the** *type* **of exercise you actually do.**

Summary:

Exercise enhances insulin sensitivity and encourages well-developed body systems, which in turn provide good health and better quality of life. **The body is developed in such a way that it functions best under conditions of regular exertion.** Once again related to feedback systems, **the body's regulatory mechanisms work optimally under the levels of physical activity common to more primitive societies.** In order to sustain this sort of 'environment' in modern times we must **simulate it through regular exercise sessions.**

This is **why** the genetic mechanisms in our bodies respond the way they do to regular exercise and to intermittent fasting. I am hopeful that the logic and information provided in this handbook will have adequately convinced you that IF is the way forward for better health and better physical appearance. **The outcomes of IF are scientific fact.**

The biggest challenge for many of us, who've been 'brainwashed' by the mainstream media and supplement promotional companies, is overcoming the perception that anything involving the word "fasting" should be avoided at all costs. I personally have had to break free of this 'conventionalist mentality' and I only managed to do so (after many years of research) because of the fact that I realised there were a large number of untested fallacies in physical culture – some of which made adherence to a healthy lifestyle a real test of determination. Many of these fallacies have been overthrown by newer, more revolutionary methodologies (through the proof of their superior or equivalent efficacy) and I believe IF will be yet another simplified solution for overcoming the lifestyle challenges of modern life.

I've used the same elimination process to totally transform my eating and exercise/sports training programs and **the results have been phenomenal** because I now get considerably better results from much less time and effort. And the results are **more predictable** than I'd get using conventional methods. Many informed people around the world are starting to do this, shouldn't you?

To discover the effectiveness of IF for health and appearance purposes one has to try it **with an open mind**. The easiest way to adapt to an IF regime is to **gradually** break it into your week - so there is actually little risk involved and potentially little to lose if you try IF on just one or two days of your week. Your muscles will not suddenly break down (in the way the 'bodybuilding and supplements crowd' used to suspect - or still claim) and you will not be overcome by unbearable, intense hunger (in the way the uniformed imagine would befall anyone who simply misses a meal).

Good luck with your journey into the modern age!

About The Author

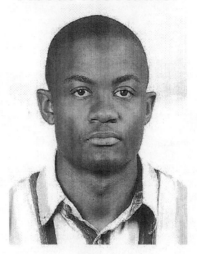

Idai Makaya is a freelance writer with a special interest in fitness conditioning, personal development and self-improvement. Qualified in Biology, Chemistry and Business Studies, Idai has a wealth of real-world life experience gained through working in many of the world's largest Healthcare corporations, at a senior level. He first became a National Manager in one of the world's largest multinational pharmaceutical organisations at just 26 years of age. Thus, he has had to find new ways of utilising his time effectively to balance family, business, fitness and other goals since then – which has led to the development of many of his fitness and health philosophies.

Idai has written a regular column on Physical Conditioning for Martial Arts Illustrated Magazine (Britain's leading Martial Arts publication) for a number of years - and has been involved in various forms of fitness training and martial arts, for most of his life. He trains in different martial arts and is ranked at Black Belt level in Tae kwon-do.

He considers himself a life-long student of self-improvement, mind, body and spiritual matters and is in the constant process of learning about life – adjusting and re-adjusting his perceptions in accordance with any new evidence which comes to light in his search.

Idai believes people exist for a purpose and part of that purpose is to make the most of every opportunity to better the world and society they live in. In order to have a positive effect on those around us, he feels we need to start by working within ourselves. Positive physical changes can lead to positive mental and spiritual changes in us (the reason, Idai believes, why many Religions and creeds rely on physical rituals as part of the strengthening of the mind and spirit). Fasting, as outlined in this book, is one such ritual which has been shown to have a lot more scientific benefit than was previously thought.

It has been said that a sound body allows for a sound mind – and for this reason Idai believes it is essential that we make the best of our health and get the most out of the bodies we live in.

Idai says *"All human life on Earth relates to and is sustained by - at least in part - the physical being. So if we are not in full control of the physical aspects of ourselves, we will probably struggle to master the more challenging psychological and spiritual aspects of our lives.*

"Take the example of being very ill. If you are unwell, it is very difficult to focus your mind on other aspects of your life - as you become preoccupied with your physical challenges. This is why it is important to maintain the best state of health possible - so you are able to free your mind to focus on positive, progressive activities.

"The principles of mastering physical discipline will be similar to those for mastering the discipline required to succeed in other forms of endeavour.

"This book is designed to help people manage their physical and, hence, psychological well-being - in order to become the best that they can be in all the different areas of their lives."

Idai Makaya lives in England with his wife, daughter and son. He believes in God and respects all the world's major religions.

Made in the USA
Lexington, KY
02 March 2011